Ama Fleud-Floyd

General Psyche Relativity Theory

***

Book 19

***

Doctrine of Psychology

***

***

Doctrine of gP/S and iP/S Therapy

***

To God, My Parents and the World

***

To My Beloved Parents –

They showed me the everlasting Pattern of Humanity.

***

***

„And the greatest of them is Love"

***

***

***

Here starts as the last of all the sciences the science of psyche.

***

***

***

The true science starts with a definition of the object of its studies. Pseudoscience gives a story, more or less interesting, but no definition.

There are millions of books and works dealing with the psyche and its disorders. Have you ever met in any of them a definition of the psyche? A valid all over the world definition?

The rest is silence?

Decide, after you read all the books of this work.

***

***

***

Definition

The Psyche is a *process* of a current symbolic *exchange* between the subject of the psyche and its current environment (subjective definition).

The Psyche is a *process* of a current symbolic *exchange* between two subjects of the psyche (objective definition).

***

***

***

Preface

I

1.

Looking at the life of wild animals, I am always amazed by their survival power. Whether in Siberian frosts or in the tropics, not to mention temperate zones, all animals are so perfectly harmonized with the Nature that they hardly ever get sick throughout their lives. They get sick only in the old age, and that is what the old age in the animals is.

2.

Meanwhile, the man as the only species among mammals is an extremely delicate species in terms of health and therefore suffers from any disease and constantly throughout the life. Why? What for? What's the point of that?

3.

It seems that we must seek the answer to this question in the very origins of the human species. I have already described them quite extensively in my works of so far in the context of the evolution of the man's psyche. And it turns out that the man's tendency to get sick is unexpectedly closely related to the question of the human psyche!

4.

I proved many times in my work the thesis that the Nature recognized the anxiety mutation as extremely dangerous for the animals and thus the prehuman apes.

Moreover, there is an evidence that the Nature considered the anxiety mutation to be definitely catastrophic. The main reason was not the destruction of the psyche. Unexpectedly the anxiety turned out to be more dangerous for the body as for the psyche! To put it short, the destruction of the organism by the anxiety is precisely the somatosis.

Since the matter goes as far back as the primary psychosis, we will therefore use from now on the term of the primary somatosis.

5.

So what is exactly the phenomenon of primary somatosis?

II

1.

 Well, the anxiety, being in the physical sense a continuous spontaneous electromagnetic brain waves emission, through continuous stimulation of the Central and Autonomous Nervous System affects the entire body by the release of the neurotransmitters and endocrine substances into the blood.

2.

 Such a constant stimulation (except for sleep) is inevitably extremely expensive in terms of energy and this is what the

Nature does not like in the long run. The energy is priceless for the Nature and that is why the process of evolution means also fighting for a free access to the energy sources and limiting loosing it.

3.

Moreover, such a constant senseless anxiety stimulation of the whole organism disturbs the course of physiological processes of all organs and systems of the organism, especially the immune system.

4.

Therefore, the Nature did not have to activate any additional mechanism to eliminate individuals with the anxiety mutation. They eliminated themselves through increased morbidity, through the primary somatosis.

5.

In other words, primary somatosis is a continuous process, triggered by the anxiety, the process of disturbing the physiological functions of the body leading to a decrease in the organism immunity and consequently to a disease.

III

1.

Contrary to the absurd theses of some psychological circles the disease has never been and will never be a "way of expression and communication". In the psychical sense illness is a completely nonsensical phenomenon and giving it any psychological meanings is an expression of a total fairy-tale writing, so readily practiced in the non-scientific field of the so-called psychology of so far.

2.

The human organic diseases are the first consequence of the anxiety. They are the physical consequence of the anxiety and from the very beginning they were supposed to eliminate the anxiety individuals from the race of evolution and the further history of life on Earth.

And there were conditions for these individuals to actually disappear as a result of the plague of diseases that befell them.

The mechanism of primary somatosis is a trap with no way out: the anxiety disturbs the physiological processes of the whole organism and as a result its immunity decreases.

3.

This is why all other animals hardly ever suffer from any diseases, living in extreme climatic and weather conditions, often cold, hungry, overheated, etc. ... The physiological processes in their bodies are not disturbed! That is why neither rain, nor cold, nor hunger are dangerous for them!

4.

And the man is so delicate, so fragile. A few minutes in the rain and the man is sick. Someone sneezes nearby and the man is sick...

5.

By the way, let's debunk the myth of a healthy lifestyle so popular in the modern people as a way to save their health.

Indeed, avoiding all threats to human health, such as biological, chemical and physical threats would make sense and would be effective, if not for the fact that the man has a mechanism of primary somatosis embedded in the genes.

IV

1.

The fact that we are alive is not the result of a healthy lifestyle because it has no importance for the somatosis.

If so, why do we live, being actually doomed to disappear from the very beginning of our race?

There is only one explanation. There is ... a miracle behind it!

What a miracle?

The Miracle of Primary Psychosis.

2.

The primary psychosis is an idea for such an aberration of the anxiety psyche so that this psyche could come out of the anxiety overload, before the evolution developed the consciousness so strong that the consciousness was able to overcome the anxiety. But before the primary psychosis the phenomenon of the somatosis appeared in the course of the evolution as the first consequence of the anxiety.

3.

Meanwhile, somatosis is the same aberration in the functioning of the human body as the psychosis in the case of the human psyche is! In both cases we are dealing with the de-realization of the functional sense of the process.

4.

And so, in the case of primary psychosis the psychological process becomes so unreal, i.e. detached from the reality that the psyche moves to a higher than real level of functioning, to a symbolic level. At this level the anxiety is deprived of the catastrophic harmfulness of its physical dimension and in the symbolic dimension the anxiety becomes a factor that inspires a creative symbolic life.

5.

What about somatosis? Here the real physiological process is replaced by an unreal, non-physiological process, i.e. a process defined by medicine as a disease process. We can therefore justifiably see an analogy between the unreal process called the disease process of the body functions and the unreal process called the psychosis of the psyche functions.

While the psychosis turns out to be an extremely valuable achievement for the human species, as it opens a new dimension of existence- the symbolic dimension; the question of whether somatosis also makes sense is extremely risky.

Let's put it clearly. All human diseases are nothing but somatoses!

And a disease process of every disease is nothing else but a detached from the physiological reality function of a given organ of the body. And even in the case of an exogenous disease the influence of an external factor is limited to inducing the derealisation of the physiological process and therefore to the same what we are dealing in an endogenous disease with. So the analogy between psyche and somatics is perfect!

Doctrine

I

1.

Let's be straightforward, many people consider P/S people not only disabled but also defective... And secretly nearly everyone thinks they are so... Until either yourself or someone from your family one day has a psyche problem... But then it's already too late. To late to claim to be treated as a normal citizen. Because the voice from the psychiatry is the voice from the world of "crazy people".

2.

The disregard for the mentally disturbed people, especially those suffering from P/S is also the reason why psychiatry has not lived to see the reliable and true drugs.

3.

When an epidemic breaks out, vaccines are ready and effective treatments developed within few years at the latest.

Meanwhile, not an epidemic, but a P/S pandemic has been going on for hundreds of years now and what a civilized modern state has managed to work out to cure millions of people from suffering? The anti-anxiety drugs. Is it a serious and dignified treatment for the P/S people?

4.

Therefore, the therapy of people suffering from P/S must start with ourselves, the so-called mentally healthy or still mentally healthy people.

5.

First, a great never-ending education of societies is needed. Starting from the kindergartens, ending with the nursing homes, going through the schools of all levels, the unions and social organizations, the religious and sports unions, it is necessary to educate everywhere to understand the mental suffering, especially the P/S suffering as the suffering that does not take away even a shadow of the right to a reliable therapy and an equal treatment.

II

1.

Secondly, hospitals and psychiatric wards as places particularly sensitive to the treatment of P/S people must set an example of dignity in treating these people, and most importantly every doctor and every medical staff must strive to ensure the reliable therapy.

2.

Third, then, therapy! Reliable therapy. Not counter-effective but effective therapy!

Well yes, but since there are still no drugs that would remove the cause of P/S and thus eliminate anxiety-free periods, how to treat?

3.

Undoubtedly, the only possible reliable therapy for genetically determined P/S is an adaptive therapy. Thus, a therapy consisting in acquiring the ability to live and to live a normal life in the society, despite the difficulties in mental functioning.

4.

The sleepy counterpart of PSPM, i.e. SSPM, often competes on the verge of sleep and waking with SPM. And this is no problem, except when the SSPM is in a nightmare setting. Nevertheless, the mankind has developed an adaptation to the competitive situation between the SSPM and the SPM. And the same, that is, the ability to adapt to the competition between PSPM and SPM should be achieved by the people with a genetic P/S disorder.

5.

Obviously, before we start such an adaptive therapy of the P/S people with the genetically determined P/S disorder they must be separated from people with P/S syndrome which appeared due to the use of anxiety blocking substances.

III

1.

Many people with induced P/S syndrome have been treated so far as people with a genetic P/S. This is a terrible mistake that must be erased first on the blame list of the psychiatry and the psychology to date. The induced P/ S from the genetic P/S to distinguish, as I described in this paper, is not difficult at all! It is enough to talk carefully with the patient and the patient's family.

2.

Only genetically P/S patients gP/S require P/S adaptive therapy. Patients with the induced P/S syndrome iP/S should leave psychiatry as soon as possible and discontinue all drugs treatment because the longer they are "treated" as gP/S, the greater the risk of psychiatrisation. In other words, after the initial period of rebellion many of them will adapt to the role of chronic mentally disturbed people. Thus, psychiatry is also a process of patient adaptation, but in the opposite direction than the reliable medicine should promote.

3.

This is because out of helplessness in front of the system a poorly diagnosed young man surrenders and adapts to the role that the system imposes. Unfortunately, this is another of the faults of the current psychiatry. Terrible guilt, with millions of broken lives.

4.

IP/S patients should be covered by the civilized State in the Program of Return to Normal Life PRNL. Their place is not a psychiatric hospital. And the damage made by the psychiatry should be stopped as soon as possible. There is a need for a process of gradual recovery of social competences. And such a program should be implemented by the state non-hospital institutions.

5.

The mentally disturbed people are a powerful army who can work for this country in all its aspects, and often quite quickly. Depending on a degree of the psychiatrisation iP/S people may regain social competences enabling normal participation in social functioning within 2 years at the latest.

IV

1.

 In the case of the gP/S people, of course, before they could go to the PRNL, they would have to undergo the process of the said P/S adaptive therapy in cooperation with the mother psychiatric hospitals and then the psychiatric outpatient clinics.

2.

 When conducting such a therapy one must bear in mind the fact that for the majority of the gP/S people the anxiety-free periods are not periods of mental suffering at all! Let us notice, because this term has been used many times here, but probably was not understood with all its consequences, namely, that there is nothing more pleasant in human life than the absence of the anxiety!

3.

So the gP/S person kind of prefers the anxiety-free periods to the normal, anxious ones! Hence, a great difficulty in the real therapy of the gP/S people. The real therapy could take away what is a blessing for them - anxiety-free periods. But those among them who are veterans of psychiatry know very well that such an effective therapy does not exist.

4.

In the contrary! The current psychiatry, by extending the anxiety-free periods with the use of anxiolytic drugs meets the hidden aspirations of gP/S patients who do not want to change anything.

5.

And this is a significant difference between gP/S and iP/S patients. For iP/S patients do not have genetically determined anxiety-free periods and they do not have this secret desire to stay as they are.

V

1.

IP/S people on the contrary! In view of the poor possibilities to develop the anti-anxiety arsenal, the obvious poverty in hospital conditions, these people are consumed by the anxiety and enormous, enormous desire to overcome this situation. Unfortunately, if they are misdiagnosed and treated like gP/S people, they are being "calmed down" by increasing doses of anti-anxiety medications. What's more, psychiatrists functioning without any scientific doctrine consider these patients as particularly dangerous to themselves and to the environment. What an irony! They consider their P/S syndrome to be extremely deep and resistant, requiring many, many years of the "therapy"...

2.

Thus, a terrible paradox is happening in psychiatric hospitals all over the world. A tragedy of a multi-million scale which the world like the Auschwitz tragedy during the war does not know or does not want to know about.

The tragedy is that in the closed wards, often in the solitary confinement, they stay for several dozen years, until they give up! And the healthy people will be forced to accept playing the role of mentally sick...

3.

Yes, healthy at least for the first years, before the system and "drugs" break their health.

4.

And in open wards or in social housing outside hospitals there are gP/S patients eagerly and meticulously accepting the anxiety therapy offered to them.

5.

Sometimes they will create a conflict situation which is understandable because during the anxiety-free periods there is no brake in the behavior, even the most ridiculous, especially when inspired by PSPM. Then they go back to the psychiatric hospitals, where everything will be done so that they can continue undisturbed to enjoy the bliss of their anxiety-free periods.

VI

1.

This is how the current system works. Globally.

2.

Yes, there is some kind of humanitarianism in the fact that people with gP/S have a possibility to live without the need to take the trouble of normal, family, professional and social existence.

3.

Or is it a distorted humanitarianism? The more distorted that at the same time millions of iP/S people are forced to stay in the psychiatric hospitals in the name, well, in the name of pseudoscience. Would a real honest science allow this?

4.

No! The theses of this book are a preview of this.

5.

So, in the P/S adaptive therapy the most important and the most difficult task is to motivate a gP/S person to leave a blissful, almost completely anxiety-free life. I note that in the anxiety-free periods it is by definition free of the anxiety, in the anxiety periods however is also anxiety-free because of the erroneous psychiatric paradigm that combats anxiety periods with the "drugs" used in P/S.

VII

1.

Of course, gP/S patients unlike iP/S patients are eager to take these drugs because what could you want more than more and more anxiety-free bliss?

2.

The lack of a scientific theory of the psyche has led to the absurd situation in which doctors become unconsciously dealers of the psychoactive substances, having no scientific vision of the psyche and its disorders. But, unfortunately, psychoactive not in the sense of restoring a gP/S person to the normal functioning, but on the contrary- there is always a progressive degradation of all social competences of the gP/S people.

3.

Nevertheless, they continue with stubbornness probably resulting only from helplessness to fight the anxiety, seeing in it the greatest enemy of the psyche. Until the complete disappearance of all higher mental functions, until a patient turns into a vegetative man. Yes, an anxiety-free man, but at the same time a man who made out of the medical staff only the suppliers of anxiolytics by dictating to doctors for decades what to do (prescribing anti-anxiety drugs, of course)

4.

Well, the system apart from the constant supply of such substances, ensures a minimum subsistence level!

5.

What an incredible system based on psychiatric-psychological pseudoscience! But let us notice that the system itself is also the evidence of the lack of any scientific foundation.

VIII

1.

In a world that does not support any vacuum, how long could such a system be not abused or even completely used? The system which is naively and carelessly providing anxiolytic substances for free and, in addition, ensuring a minimum subsistence level for all recipients of the state dealer?

2.

It is an unbelievable thing that a naive legislator donates mountains of money to make out of the state the biggest dealer of psychoactive substances. Naive because the legislature has no idea of the fact that the system is based on a scientific void. How is the legislature to know this? From the thousands of psychiatry professors?

3.

Why not? Could there not be a single honest among thousands of psychiatry professors who would admit that the psychiatry professorship is a fiction because you cannot be a professor of pseudoscience?

4.

No, that's not the reason. The "professors" of psychiatry are just as honest as professors of all other fields of science. The thing is about something else.

5.

 Now, you don't become a professor in recognition of your merits in search of the truth. Unfortunately not. Although maybe someone believes it...

IX

1.

The professors are produced. The universities produce them. And why do the universities produce professors?

It is obvious, without them the university cannot earn money in educating students.

2..

And what do professors teach their students? They teach what was and what is. After all, you cannot teach what will be.

3.

In other words, university professors are guardians of the existing state of the knowledge and of the ignorance of science, making sure that all erroneous theories of the past are passed on to the next generation of "scholars"...

4.

Despite the university and its professors, the science, the real science develops outside of universities. Yes, but it has to be science not pseudoscience.

5.

The pseudoscience, inside or outside academia, is still pseudoscience. Hence, the tragedy of psychiatry. It is a pseudoscience.

X

1.

In my earlier books, I have clarified this point. As a reminder, let me just say that the real science can define the subject of its research. And that's all it takes to be science. Only and so much...

2.

Unfortunately, the current psychiatry and psychology cannot do even that much. Because what kind of psychology (or the science of the psyche) is this, if this "science" has not worked out the cornerstone of every, even the most modest science, that is, the definition of the subject of its research. In XXI century there is all the time no scientific definition of the psyche!

3.

Excuse me. It has not existed so far. This and my other works change that.

4.

So, the most important thing in the P/S therapy is to separate people falsely diagnosed as gP/S. Then, the real gP/S must be passed through the P/S adaptive therapy.

5.

 As I wrote earlier, most gP/S patients succumb to the demoralizing impact of psychiatry and repairing this massive anomaly will require fundamental changes to the entire psychiatric care system.

XI

1.

The gP/S patient should never again, with the overactive participation of the state, find himself in the niche of a disorder, making out of it the only "occupation" throughout his life.

2.

The P/S adaptive therapy already at the hospital stage and then in the preparatory and adaptation institutions must teach to leave the P/S niche, to go to work, to go to everyday life, the life of all citizens. P/S disorder shouldn't be a reason for the patient to be marginalized. It should not be an excuse for resignationism.

3.

The P/S adaptive therapy is the most important strategy of fighting P/S disorder. As I wrote before, there is no and never will be a miracle pill that will cure them.

4.

Another fault of the current psychiatry, perhaps the greatest one, is that the "drugs" administered to P/S patients are presented as drugs treating this disorder. As I have broadly justified it, this is not true.

5.

Of course, it is difficult to accept the truth which I am proclaiming here. Namely, the truth that pharmacological treatment of P/S is impossible. This, no doubt, is a great disappointment and pain for millions of people and their families. Especially families. However, it is a great consolation for troubled people, when they can hope that what has happened to them or their loved ones can be treated with a pill...

XII

1.

But it is precisely this hope that I am trying to save! I believe it is possible to treat P/S with the P/S adaptive therapy!

2.

Yes, I do give up hope as to the "drugs" currently used in P/S. In my opinion, the false hope is much worse than the not-so-delicious truth that not the drug therapy, but only adaptive therapy is the only reliable and sensible form of the P/S treatment.

3.

 Wishing you maybe a successful therapy one day or just understanding the groundbreaking nature of this General Psyche Relativity Theory in the history of your struggles with your own psyche.

Exordium

***

***

Definition

The Psyche is a *process* of a current symbolic *exchange* between the subject of the psyche and its current environment (subjective definition).

The Psyche is a *process* of a current symbolic *exchange* between two subjects of the psyche (objective definition).

✳✳✳

✳✳✳

✳✳✳

I

1.

In my work I explain this definition. My definition of the psyche defines it as a dynamic phenomenon. Not static one as the psyche was understood and described untill now.

2.

In other words all static descriptions of the psyche are only metaphors. It means that in reality all the psychology language of so far, starting with Freud's works and millions of books of other authors, should be seen as kind of poetry and not, of course, as a scientific writing! However, it has been understood untill now literally! And in such a way a false science misled the civilization and millions of suffering people.

3.

Meanwhile, it is an absurd that such an obvious to everybody statement sounds like a great discovery that the psyche is not an observable object. After all, nobody has ever seen it! So we can neither observe it, nor describe it as an object.

4

This absurd is more absurd than the situation before Copernicus regarding the obvious common observation that the Sun moved on the sky. Everybody could see it with his own eyes. And still Copernicus was the only one to question this common observation.

5.

As a matter of fact it was the declaration of Copernicus what was absurd! In a way, being contradictory to the observable fact, the declaration of Copernicus was in a justified way rejected by the science of that time. The science before Him had an observable proof of what moved and what did not. Still the final proof could get only those of us who could see the Earth from the cosmic space. It means that the observation, being a basis of all science, is not however enough to be decisive. The point of view of the observation is decisive.

II

1.

The surface of the Earth was a wrong point of view to decide, if the Sun moved around the Earth or was it the other way round. But untill XX century it was the only accessible point of view, so untill cosmic trips the observation that the Sun moves around the Earth was totally justifiable.

2.

With my work I want to show that in the case of the psyche it is also the question of the point of view.

3.

Untill now the psychology was founded on the static point of view on the psyche. The psyche was described by Freud, the founder of the XX century psychology, as a static object. It was devided by him in a typically static way in portions, like: „ego", „superego", „id", „consiousness", „subconsciousness". It was a kind of a magic world with its enigmatic static structures, a world of objects totally strange to an every day life of the people. And hence, the necessity of a translator which a psychotherapist is supposed to be. It is assumed by a client that the psychotherapist knows the enigmatic world of the psyche and will be able to describe it in a language understood by everybody.

This approach resembles a lot the way the spiritual groups function like. Both in the case of the psychology of so far and in the case of spiritual groups there is a group of people who „know" the „sacred" knowledge about respectively the psyche and the spiritual world and there is the rest of the people who know nothing or know only as much as those who „know" will tell them. Two worlds: sacrum (the world where only those who know have an access to) and profanum (the clients of those who know).

5.

Actually, what is this „sacred" knowledge of the psychology of so far?

It is an invented and all the time anew reinvented story about the sacrum- an enigmatic world of the psyche, where nothing is certain, everything possible, and the most important role is played by those who „know" to tell a client a story about the psyche.

III

1.

The biggest of the storytellers of the psychology of so far, like Freud, were those whose stories were the most original and... strange. Why strange? Because the „sacrum" cannot be as banal as the „profanum", if they should be clearly separated from each other. Without this separation there would be no need for those who „know". This explains why „psychology" of so far has not come untill now to became a science.

2.

The science is a destroyer of the sacrum, because the science discovers the laws to understand the world. And the world governed by the laws is no longer enigmatic. In this way the sacrum becomes the profanum. In consequence those who „know" are superfluous. Knowing the laws of the Nature and using logical thinking is enough to get on in the profanum world. Everybody can do it.

3.

This is why those who „know" in the „psychology" of so far are the last to try to establish and popularize any laws ruling the psyche (if they happen to discover them). A day, when the psyche becomes the science, will be their last day. They will combat before, however, any real attempt to make the psychology become the science.

4.

When it comes to the psyche, everybody from his own experience accepts the fact that it exists. The question is only that nobody could ever see it with the eyes as an observable object. Nevertheless everybody accepts its metaphorical descriptions as if they were those of an observable object. Why?

5.

Because untill now people have had no choice! The same as untill Copernicus. There was no alternative. People believe in what authors write. You get to your hands the alternative to the description of the psyche of so far.

IV

1.

So, what can we say about the psyche? Scientifically speaking, only this what can be observed. Of course, as the example of Copernicus shows, observation itself is not a guarantee that what we see is what we see. But in the case of the psyche it is just the reverse of the case of Copernicus. Because the observation of so far sees nothing!

2.

Untill cosmic trips scientific procedure based on the observation, which is the condition sine qua non of the true science, could not accept the calculations of Copernicus. Even if mathematically speaking they looked correct and plausible. In other words Copernicus, 400 years before the observation made from the point of view of the cosmic space, gave mathematical arguments that the observation made from the point of view of the Earth surface was wrong.

3.

My role in the history of the psyche exploration is the reverse of the role played by Copernicus in the cosmos exploration.

4.

Namely, Copernicus with mathematical arguments proved that the description of the *observation* of the Sun movement on the sky was only a guise of the true. And the mistake of that false observation consisted in a wrong point of view of the observation of the Sun movement.

5.

I, in turn, with my logics, biology, physics, chemistry and evolutionary arguments try to prove that the description of the psyche in force based on *no observation* is also only a guise of the true. A guise which is the same invented as it was before Copernicus.

V

1.

One thing jumps however to the eyes. People 2000, 1000 and 400 years ago seemed to be better thinkers than people today! Why?

These ancient people, even if wrong in their description of the Sun movement, are excused by the argument of the *observation* in their favor.

People of the XX century, in turn, believe in a description of the psyche based on the argument of *no observation*...

2.

My role in this turning point of the psyche exploration is to stop the era of descriptions of the psyche based on no observation. In order to make this observation possible I had to search for a possibility to observe the psyche. And this possibility could be found, but not there where millions and millions of people have not found it before me. It could not be found in the static dimension of the reality.

3.

My Copernican breakthrough was to move my point of view of the psyche observation from the *static* dimension of the reality to the *dynamic* one. And this act made all the difference. I could finally *observe* and *define*, what the psyche is. Definition of the psyche in hand, I could start the science of the psyche.

4.

And what can be observed is a dynamic phenomenon. The dynamic process!

This dynamic process I call in my definition of the psyche- the current symbolic exchange! It means that it is not possible to talk about the psyche of a person. It does not exist. What exists is only the psyche as a momentary current symbolic exchange. It means that the psyche of a person is a sequence of infinitely small momentary symbolic exchanges, the same as the light is the sequence of infinitely small fotons of light.

For this reason the psyche as a process can be disturbed, but, of course, can not be sick (!) and for this reason (not the only one) the title of this work is:

„General Psyche *Relativity* Theory".

5.

(Of course, you will still find in this work expressions reminding of the era of the static psyche descriptions (two poles, inter-polar space,...).

I could not, however, start writing about the psyche using the language which is not understood by you, my dear Reader, already from the first pages. For a very simple reason: nobody before me wrote about the psyche as about a dynamic phenomenon, like the light or the time.

You maybe wonder, why I am the only one to treat the psyche as a phenomenon and not like an object. The answer is easy. Because I have never seen the psyche and I have never heard that anybody has. Still, it exists! The conclusion is one: it is a dynamic phenomenon.)

Abbreviations

AB Anxiety Blocker

AEA Anxiety-Emotional Alertness

AEI Anxiety-Emotional Intelligence

CP Cyclic Polysymbolicity

CS Childishness Syndrome

EP Episodic Psychosis

ESE External Self-Esteem

ESEx External Symbolic Exchange

gP/S genetic Polysymbolicity/Schizophrenia

iP/S Induced Polysymbolicity/Schizophrenia

ISE Internal Self-Esteem

ISEx Internal Symbolic Exchange

LI Logic Intelligence

NPP Negative Primary Psychosis (Depression)

PSPM Parallel Symbolic Psyche Me

PRNL Program of Return to Normal Life

PSEx Parallel Symbolic Exchange

SBM Symbolic Brain Me

SE Self-Esteem

SEx Symbolic Exchange

SP Simultaneous Polysymbolicity

SPM Symbolic Psyche Me

SSPM Sleep Symbolic Psyche Me

T1h Type 1 of the Humanity (without self-distance to the primary psychosis)

T2h Type 2 of the Humanity (with self-distance to the primary psychosis)

T3h Type 3 of the Humanity (intermidate type between T1h and T2h)

www.ingramcontent.com/pod-product-compliance
Lightning Source LLC
Chambersburg PA
CBHW070446220526
45466CB00004B/1775